Hair Growing Magic Potion

20 Natural Homemade Hair Care Recipes That Guarantees Long and Fast Hair Growth

MOIRA GLENWOOD

ISBN-13: 978-1530039432

ISBN-10: 1530039436

DEDICATION

To all who desire to live life to the fullest!

TABLE OF CONTENT

INTRODUCTION

As a beauty activist and "all things natural" enthusiast, author, mother and wife. Years ago I had issues with my hair growth; I was exhausted, unhappy and desperately aching for a better length of hair. One day, gruelingly tired of my situation, I started researching everything I could on hair growth and transforming the length of my hair. I soon found out and decided to share with you in very clear straight to the point terms.

Are you like me and you are starting to think more of natural hair, with a good shine that also grows well lately? Or probably you have been natural for many years but sometimes you still feel like you don't have your routine down? Are you tired of store bought natural hair products that don't seem to give your hair enough of the moisture and desired growth needed or define your curls?

This book has a list of natural homemade recipes that you can create yourself to use in your natural hair care routine. You made a great choice buying. Enjoy reading.

1 inch in 1 week hair growth oil

Ingredients

Your favorite oil: extra virgin or coconut olive

(Any scalp oil of your choice)

Directions

Warm about two to three tablespoons of your favorite scalp oil and massage over your scalp and hair. Bend over so that your head is completely downwards. Note: You should be looking underneath the seat you are sitting on. This is known as inversion. It reverses the blood flow to the scalp to get hair growing. Invert for five minutes while giving a scalp massage. Do the oil and inversion for Seven days and you should see good results!

Warning: if you are pregnant or unhealthy do not invert please. If you feel dizzy or light headed when inverting, DON'T DO IT.

Mustard Mask for Hair Growth

Ingredients

2 tablespoons of olive oil

2 tablespoons of ground mustard powder

1 egg yolk

2 teaspoons of sugar

2 tablespoons of hot water

Directions:

Combine water with mustard, add yolk, oil and sugar and combine very well. Part the hair into sections and put mix on the scalp. Do not put it on your hair ends. After you have applied to your hair, put on a plastic shower cap and on the top of it something warm to keep the heat in. It will heat up very quickly but that is very normal. It might start burning, but it's a good burn. But if you feel it's like an allergic reaction burn or so uncomfortable that you cannot take it, wash it out. Sit for a minimum of fifteen mins (maximum up to one hour).

After a minimum of fifteen mins, rinse the mask with warm water until the water runs and clear and then use you can use your favorite shampoo. It is advised that the mask should be done at least twice in a week for at least one or two months depending how slowly your hair grows.

Essential Growth Oil

Ingredients

½ teaspoon of jojoba oil

3 drops of lavender

2 drops of rosemary

2 drops of thyme

4 teaspoon of Grape seed oil (carrier oil)

Direction:

Combine all five ingredients well and then massage into the scalp for 2 mins. To increase absorption, wrap a warm towel around your head. With a mild shampoo, wash the hair after an hour. Make this a daily routine for at least 7 months.

Use a spray or an applicator bottle to apply to scalp as you need (on a daily basis).

The Healthy Hair Grow mixture

Ingredients

2 avacados

1 or 2 bananas (depending on the length of your hair)

2 teaspoons of shea butter

2 to 3 drops of tea tree oil

1 drop of eucalyptus oil

Directions:

You can mix or blend all ingredients together and put in a bowl. Wait until you conclude shampooing and conditioning your hair, then you distribute it evenly into your hair. Massage effectively into your hair and scalp. Then comb your hair with a wide tooth comb and leave in for five to ten mins.

Rinse your hair out thoroughly.

Hair Growth Hot Oil Treatment

Ingredients such as rosemary helps to stimulate growth of hair, while it clears away of impurities and nourishing the scalp.

Ingredients

3 drops of essential oil of lavender

1/8 cup of grapeseed oil

3 drops of essential oil of rosemary

3 drops of essential oil of cedarwood

1/8 cup of jojoba oil

3 drops of essential oil of thyme

Directions

Combine all six ingredients together and then apply at night before sleeping, to your scalp in the thinning areas. Don't rinse out until it is morning.

Natural Growth Stimulating Conditioner

Ingredients:

¼ cup of plain natural yogurt

1 egg

1 teaspoon of fresh lemon juice

8 to 10 drops of eucalyptus oil (or olive oil, or rosemary oil, or rosemary/olive oil and canola oil)

Directions:

Process all the ingredients together in a blender. Massage onto and scalp hair and leave for a minimum of twenty to thirty mins before washing out.

Oil Blend for Hair Growth

Although there is no much guarantee that this blend will stimulate growth, many people have reported that they noticed a difference in the length of their hair

Ingredients

1/8 cup jojoba oil

3 drops thyme essential oil

3 drops lemon essential oil

3 drops cedarwood essential oil

3 drops rosemary essential oil

3 drops lavender essential oil

1/8 cup grapeseed oil

Directions

Combine all seven ingredients together in a small bowl, and place in a bottle. Shake well and then apply several drops of the mixture to your scalp and other areas of hair loss each night, massaging gently into your scalp for three to five mins. Store the oil tightly covered and kept away from heat and light.

Note: A pregnant woman should avoid rosemary essential oil.

ACV Growth Rinse

This hair growth portion is perfect as a final rinse and helps to promote and enhance hair growth. Rosemary has been used for several hundreds of years as a scalp stimulator.

Ingredients:

2 Tablespoons of Rosemary Dried Leaf

1 cup of Apple Cider Vinegar

1 cup of water

Directions

Place the rosemary in vinegar. Microwave the mixture for thirty seconds. Spoon the leaves that remained from the vinegar on the side of the jar. Strain the vinegar with the smallest available strainer you can lay your hands on (I recommend cut up pantyhose) and then add water. Apply as a final rinse.

Coconut and Honey Cooling Hair Mask

Ingredients:

Castor oil

Avocado oil

Peppermint essential oil

Olive oil

Raw honey

Shea Moisture Raw Shea Butter Deep Treatment Masque

Organic Coconut Milk

Directions:

Mix in the castor, honey, olive and avocado oils together. Stir until it becomes smooth. Mix the Shea moisture deep conditioning mask and coconut milk together. Stir until it becomes smooth.

Add the oil and honey mix to the coconut milk and Shea moisture mix stir until it becomes smooth. The mixture should be creamy and thick.

If you want additional scalp stimulation add ten to twenty drops of peppermint essential oil drops to the final mixture. Apply the mix to a clean and freshly washed hair. Leave on for a minimum of thirty minutes. Rinse with cool water.

Coconut Milk & Oil Recipe for Shiny Waves

This conditioning mixture is good when you want your curls moisturized. It works perfectly on normal, dry or oily hair. It strengthens your hair and adds shine to it, so it's also good for correcting hair loss and enhancing hair growth.

Ingredients

1 tablespoon of your favorite hair conditioner (you can use Senscience's Inner

Restore Intensif masque... but your choice matters)

1 tablespoon of Cane molasses

3 tablespoon of Coconut milk (or add to taste)

1 tablespoon of Coconut Oil

1 tablespoon of Honey

1 tablespoon of Rosemary infused Olive oil (or just plain olive oil)

Directions:

Combine ingredients manually in a small bowl or on a mixer, whatever works for you. Divide your hair into 4 sections and apply mixture from roots of your hair to the hair ends on every section, massaging the hair portion as you apply the mixture.

Do not rinse out immediately, you should leave it on for a minimum of an hour or for as long as you wish. Apply it on your hair that is pre-shampooed or second or third day hair (make sure it's still very clean).

Note: You can substitute the olive oil for any other oil of your choice.

Caribbean Smoothie

This hair growth portion leaves your hair silky, smooth and soft and also strong and very healthy. It also helps with rapid hair growth!

Ingredients

Note: ingredients can be tweaked, depending on the length of hair.

½ avocado (ripe)

½ cup of Coconut milk

½ banana (ripe)

1 tablespoon of Castor oil

2 tablespoon of Rosemary

1 teaspoon of Cayenne Pepper

Directions:

Combine all six ingredients in a blender, and process until it becomes smooth. Then apply the mixture from the ends of your hair to the roots and massage it in. Leave in for fifteen minutes to one hour. Rinse out completely with warm water.

Protein Humectant Deep Conditioner

This wonderful hair growth portion, PHDC retains moisture and it also adds protein to the hair –those are 2 key factors in hair growth and strength!

Ingredients

5 drops peppermint oil

1/4C extra virgin olive oil

1 egg

1/8C honey

1 avocado

1 teaspoon of biotin powder

Directions:

Combine all six ingredients together until it has a consistency that looks batter-like. Apply a generous amount to dry or damp hair. Cover your hair with a plastic cap or towel or both towel and plastic cap and/or sit under a dryer. Let the conditioner sit for thirty mins to one hour. Rinse with cool water.

Aloe Vera and Oil Shampoo

This hair growth is anti-fungal, anti-bacterial and hair growth promoting

Ingredients:

Water

Aloe Vera gel (better if it's fresh)

essential oils (rosemary, olive, castor, canola....)

Directions:

Blend some of the aloe Vera gel and ¼ or ½ of a cup of water and an essential oil of your choice (olive or rosemary or castor oil). Process in a blender till it becomes smooth and then pour into a container

Mayo Deep Treatment

This treatment is full of moisturizing agents, protein and more. You should use this treatment as a deep conditioning treatment to quench the thirst in your curls! it also helps to promote the growth of hair.

Ingredients:

3 tablespoons Honey

4 drops of Peppermint EO

4 tablespoons of Real Mayo

EVOO

1 Egg

EVCO

4 drops of Rosemary EO

Directions

Combine all seven ingredients together, mix thoroughly. And then apply to your hair after shampooing. Leave on for a minimum of one hour. Rinse well with cool water.

Homemade Leave-in Conditioner

This recipe promotes hair growth, prevents hair loss, prevents dandruff, cleanses the hair and scalp, prevents dry and itchy scalp, among many other things it does.

Ingredients:

10 small squirts of Lime Juice (naturally cleanses the hair and scalp, removes hair odors, prevents dandruff)

½ cup of Aloe Juice and gel (great for hair loss, a natural conditioner, great for dry and itchy scalps)

1 cup purified water

Milk/Water from 1 coconut

1 tablespoon of melted Shea butter, vitamin E (decreases sun damage, promotes growth, antioxidant)

1tablespoon of melted Coconut Oil

1 teaspoon of Olive oil (prevents dandruff and moisturizes)

½ teaspoon of Thyme oil (gives natural shine, promotes healthy scalp and prevents hair loss)

1teaspoon of Rosemary oil (prevents hair loss, promotes growth, moisturizes and prevents dandruff)

Directions:

Combine all ingredients together and blend until it becomes smooth. When it is finely blended, transfer into a spray bottle.

Protein Deep Conditioner with Castor Oil

I started using this recipe about two months ago and I really love it for my hair. It is a simple recipe that consists of the usual mayonnaise and egg ingredients; but I also learnt to tweak and incorporate more ingredients

Ingredients:

1 tbsp of mayonnaise

1 egg

1 tsp of cold pressed castor oil

1-2 tsps of olive oil

1 drop of vitamin E oil

1 tbsp of rinse out conditioner (if desired, just in case may want some extra moisture)

Note: You can decide to double the ingredients if you have a lot of hair length. In the making of this recipe, the amount of ingredients that was used is for a twelve inches long hair or lesser.

Directions:

Combine all ingredients well in an empty bowl until it becomes well blended.

Divide your hair into sections for better distribution and apply to washed hair. Work the conditioner into each separate section.

Make sure you saturate your hair well!

Cover your hair with a plastic cap and leave on for twenty to thirty mins (You can also choose to sit under a dryer or heated cap for half the time); Rinse and wash out using your regular rinse out conditioner!

Note: you can use any essential oil that catches your fancy to trap the moisture. Feel the softness of your hair. Hope you like it!

Ayurvedic mask

This is a protein ayurvedic mud mask that is certain to send your curls poppin. This recipe certainly strengthens any coil, curl or kink back into shape and provides long lasting elasticity. The Brahmi in the ingredients promotes growth of hair

Ingredients:

Aloe vera juice or Coconut Milk

Ayurvedic henna mixture which includes Brahmi, hibiscus powder, shikakai, aloe vera, amla, bhringraj, neem, and jatamansi powders. You can use Nupur henna gotten from most local indian stores which includes all this in one package.

Your favorite moisture rinse out conditioner

One large egg

Coconut oil

Agave nectar or Honey

Directions

It depends on the hair type; in a plastic bowl, place 1-2 full cups of Nupur henna powder. Place one cup of aloe vera juice or coconut milk to one cup of henna mixture or one and half cup of aloe vera juice or coconut milk to two cups henna mixture. Place a 1 ½ tbsp of coconut oil in one cup of henna mixture or 2 1/3 of coconut oil to two cups henna mixture. Add a large egg to the mixture.

2 tbsps of honey or agave nectar to 1 cup of henna mixture or 4 table spoons to 2 cups henna mixture.

Finally add one cup of your favorite moisture rinse out conditioner to one cup of henna mixture or two cups to two cups of henna mixture.

Divide your hair into sections to help even distribution, apply to hair sections and wrap with a plastic cap. Leave on for one to three hours or however long you'd like, and then rinse thoroughly with protein free moisture rich conditioner for bouncy and shiny curls then style as you would.

Allow the water from your shower head to rinse the mixture out, less bending, twisting and manipulation of the hair while the mixture is still in will prevent any tangles and knots from forming.

Coconut Oil Base Hot Oil Treatment

I just started using this hot oil treatment for my hair!

Ingredients:

(The amount of ingredients you use depends on the length and thickness of your hair! This is for short-medium length haired people)

1 tablespoons of Castor Oil

2 tablespoons of Coconut Oil

1 tablespoon of Jojoba Oil

2 drops of Vitamin E Oil

1 teaspoon of Peppermint Oil

Olive oil, optional

Directions:

Wash your hair and divide the hair into three to four sections. After your hair has been washed, combine the oils together in a jar or bowl and heat until it is warm and melted (You can heat the oils by placing the jar or bowl in boiled water, or put in a microwave for thirty to forty five seconds). Apply to your scalp and then saturate each section individually.

 Keep your plastic cap on for ten to fifteen minutes or sit under a heated dryer or hood for five to ten mins. Finally condition your hair

Pumpkin Seed Butter Mask

This butter mask has a lot of healthy benefits that most people with curls and coils desire and are always trying to incorporate into their hair regimens. This butter mask will promote curl definition and growth.

Ingredients:

2 tablespoons of Sunny Isle Jamaican Black Castor Oil Extra Dark

2 tablespoons of Dastony 100% Organic Sprouted Pumpkin Seed Butter

2 tablespoons of GPB Glycogen Protein Balancing Conditioner

Directions:

Combine equal parts of the Castor Oil, Pumpkin Seed butter and Conditioner. Apply to slightly damp or dry hair. You may need to add more conditioner for easier application on your hair...this mixture does NOT provide slip for your hair, it is a mask, so it just needs to get worked into your hair and on the strands. Wear a plastic shower cap/ plastic bag on it for a minimum of one hour. The mask will become dry stiff. Rinse and cleanse or cowash. You can use it as a pre treatment to your wash day regimen, but you can also use as a deep conditioner as well! (You should still rinse out with a favorite conditioner if you use as a dc, for detangling and to make sure the whole product has been well removed)

Natural hair growth serum

This natural hair growth serum combines essential oils and herbs that are good for hair growth and scalp health:

Nettle: the nettle is rich in vitamins A, vitamin C, vitamin K, Iron, plus magnesium and potassium. It is often used in making natural hair products and it also helps stimulate hair growth.

Horsetail: the horsetail is high in silica and excellent for the hair, as it supports hair growth.

Aloe Vera Gel: the aloevera gel naturally soothes and thickens the scalp and serves as a silkening base for this serum.

Essential Oils: Essential oils of Rosemary, Clary Sage and Lavender are great for hair and scalp health.

Where to Get Ingredients

You can get the horsetail leaf and nettle leaf from Mountain Rose Herbs and the natural aloe vera.

For the essential oils, any high quality option will work. You can order your oils from Mountain Rose Herbs, and Plant Therapy.

Ingredients

1 cup of distilled water

10 drops of Lavender Essential Oil

2 tbsps of Dried Nettle Leaf

10 drops of Rosemary Essential Oil

2 tbsps of Natural Aloe Vera Gel

10 drops of Clary Sage Essential Oil

2 tbsps of Horsetail Leaf (if desired)

Directions:

Boil the distilled water and add the horsetail leaf and dried nettle leaf. Let the herbs sit in the water for a minimum of ten mins or until the water becomes cool. Strain the herbs out and pour the herb infused liquid in to a spray bottle. Add essential oils and the aloe vera and then shake well. Store in the refrigerator for up to three months and shake well before you use.

Spray freely and generously on your hair roots once or more per day. I have found that it was easiest and worked the best to spray on before bed each night.

END

Thank you for reading my book. If you enjoyed it, won't you please take a moment to look at my other titles?

Thanks!

Nancy Crews